Free From Breast Cancer:

How to Recognize and Fight Against the Silent Killer

Dr. Edward A. Johnson

Table of contents

Introduction

The most common kind of fatal cancer among women identified globally is breast cancer. It is the greatest cause of cancer death in women in many less developed nations; in industrialized nations, however, lung cancer has surpassed it as the major cause of cancer death in women. Breast cancer is the second leading cause of cancer-related deaths in women in the United States, after lung cancer, accounting for 31% of all malignancies in females. Early breast carcinomas frequently have no symptoms; breast cancer is not typically characterized by pain or discomfort. Before it is felt by the patient or recognized by a healthcare professional, breast cancer is frequently first found as an anomaly on mammography.

Triple assessment is now the standard method for evaluating breast cancer and includes clinical examination, imaging (often mammography, ultrasonography, or both), and needle biopsy.

Early diagnosis at stages amenable to qqaacomplete surgical resection and curative treatments has been made possible by increased public awareness and enhanced screening. For women with breast cancer, improved therapy and screening have increased survival rates.

Breast cancer is today treated mostly with surgery, radiation therapy, and, if necessary, adjuvant hormone or chemotherapy. Surgery combined with local radiation therapy is curative for many individuals with low-risk early-stage breast cancer. Breast cancer cells that have exited the breast and local lymph nodes but do not yet have a confirmed detectable metastasis are treated with adjuvant therapy for breast cancer. Adjuvant therapy has been predicted to be responsible for 35-72% of the decline in mortality, depending on the risk reduction model.

Extensive and advocate-driven breast cancer research over the past three decades has greatly advanced our knowledge of the condition. This has led to the creation of less harmful and more targeted treatments.

Chapter 1

What is Breast Cancer?

Breast tissue is where breast cancer develops. It occurs when breast cells experience unchecked proliferation and change. The cells typically develop into a tumor.

Cancer may not advance in all cases. It is known as "in situ." If the cancer spreads outside the breast, it is said to be "invasive." It might have just impacted tissues and lymph nodes close by. Instead, cancer may metastasize (spread to other organs) through the blood or lymphatic system.

In the United States, breast cancer is the second most prevalent type of cancer in women. Sometimes, men may also be affected.

Breast cancer develops when a breast cell mutates and begins to divide quickly. Each year, more than 275,000 new cases of breast cancer are discovered in the US. Luckily, new therapies have increased the five-year survival rate of the illness to 90%.

Everyone has at least a modest amount of breast tissue, regardless of biological sex. Your pectoral overlies your breast (chest muscles). The breast's shape is mostly created by fatty tissue and a small amount of connective tissue. Moreover, lymph nodes—tiny, bean-shaped organs that assist in the movement of immune cells and the removal of waste from tissue—are found in the breasts. In females, the breast also contains specific glands with the ability to make milk. These glands are known as lobules, and a network of tiny tubes known as ducts connects them to the nipple.

Breast tissue cells develop into cancer when they multiply and expand out of control. Although it can also affect men, it primarily affects women. Your prognosis, treatment options, and kind of breast cancer are all influenced by several variables. These variables include the location of cancer's onset, its invasiveness, and the cancer cells' molecular receptor status.

Symptoms of breast cancer

Breast cancer symptoms differ from person to person, and the sensation of a lump or mass cannot be precisely described. Knowing your breasts well will help you understand how "normal" feels and appears. Inform your doctor of any changes you observe. While routine self-examinations are vital, frequent screening mammography can identify many breast cancers before any symptoms arise.
Breast lumps or masses are among the signs of breast cancer.
• Bulge or lump under the arm
• Breast skin changes, such as skin redness and thickness give the skin an orange-peel appearance.
• Dimpling or puckering on the breast
• Nipple discharge
• Scaliness on the nipple, which can occasionally spread to the areola
• Nipple adjustments, such as the nipple tugging inward, twisting inward, or changing directions.
• A breast or nipple ulcer that occasionally spreads to the areola

• Breast enlargement

The examination must include a review of the breasts with the patient standing erect and their arms elevated to notice minute changes in breast contour and skin tethering. The following discoveries should cause alarm:

• Edema or peau d'orange
• Skin tethering
• Skin lump or shape alteration
• Nipple inversion
• Dilated veins
• Ulceration
• Mammary Paget disease

Clinically determining the nature of palpable lumps is frequently challenging, but the following characteristics should cause concern:

•Asymmetry with the opposite breast
• focal nodularity
• hardness, and irregularities
• Fixation to muscle or skin (assess fixation to the muscle by moving the lump in the line of the pectoral muscle fibers with the patient bracing her arms against her hips)

Assessing for lymphatic and distant metastases is a crucial part of a thorough physical; in terms of frequency, distant metastases to the bone, lung, liver,
and brain are the least common. The assessment should therefore include exams of the axillae and supraclavicular fossae, the chest, the painful bone locations, the abdomen, and the nervous system. The doctor should be aware of the following signs of metastatic spread:
• Chest pain
• Hypercalcemia signs
• Respiratory issues
• Distention of the abdomen
• Localizing neurological symptoms
• Modifications in cognitive function
• Headache
It's not always the case that these symptoms indicate breast cancer. The symptoms you experience should be discussed with your doctor, though, as they could also be signs of other health issues.

Where breast cancer begins

Although breast cancer can arise in a variety of different tissue types, the majority of cases fall into one of two categories: ductal carcinomas, which begin in the ducts, or lobular carcinomas, which begin in the lobule glands. Other breast cancer kinds are listed below.

- **Invasive vs. Non-Invasive**

Depending on whether they have migrated to the surrounding tissue, invasive and non-invasive breast cancers can be further classified as a subset of lobular and ductal carcinomas. Ductal carcinoma in situ, also known as non-invasive ductal carcinoma, is a form of early-stage cancer that has not gone past the ducts. Usually, it is discovered during a normal mammography or breast check. Ductal carcinoma is regarded as invasive if it spreads to the surrounding tissue. Cancer that is diagnosed most frequently is invasive ductal carcinoma.

It is less frequent and not exactly categorized as cancer as non-invasive lobular carcinoma, also known as lobular carcinoma in situ. Having lobular carcinoma in situ, however, may increase your risk of later getting breast cancer. (For further breast cancer risk factors, see below.) If lobular carcinoma has affected nearby lymph nodes or other breast tissue, it is said to be invasive. Compared to invasive ductal carcinoma, invasive lobular carcinoma is less frequent.

Cancer cells' molecular receptor state

On the exterior of cancer cells are molecules called receptors. These receptors can interact or bind with particular proteins and hormones in the body of the sufferer. We refer to this as awareness.

Researchers have discovered specific receptors that, upon recognizing a particular molecule, promote the development and spread of breast cancer. Cancer medications can stop or slow the progression of the illness by preventing this recognition.

Currently, three main receptor subtypes are crucial to the therapy and prognosis of the patient. Additional receptor subtypes with various therapeutic options could be discovered as breast cancer research progresses. The three main subtypes follow.

1. HER2-positive breast cancer

The protein HER2, or human epidermal growth factor receptor 2, is essential for cell growth. HER2-positive breast cancers are those that have a lot of HER2 on their cancer cell surfaces. When two of these proteins bond they form a dimer, which sends a signal to the cell that promotes growth and multiplication Anti-HER2 therapy, which targets the HER2 protein, is one form of treatment. About 15%–20% of all breast cancer cases are HER2-positive.

Hormone receptor-positive/ER-positive cancers make up about half of HER2-positive cancers. Treatments for these patients focus on both molecular receptors. As HER2 is thought to be the main cause of the illness, they are categorized as HER2-positive.

A higher chance of recurrence was once linked to a HER2-positive diagnosis. The disease is now more treatable in its early stages thanks to recent advancements in medicine, especially with targeted therapies. Patients whose cancer metastasized, or had spread beyond the breast and nearby lymph nodes, have also had their survival times prolonged.

2. Breast carcinoma with ER-positive hormone receptors

The most typical form of breast cancer is hormone receptor-positive breast cancer. Receptors for this illness attach to either of the two naturally occurring hormones, progesterone or estrogen. By attaching to these receptors, these chemicals promote the development of cancer.

The growth of cancer is stopped or slowed down by endocrine therapy, also referred to as hormone therapy, which targets this receptor/hormone recognition. These treatments have the potential to reduce the body's production of estrogen and progesterone or prevent the hormones from binding to the receptors.

Hormone receptor-positive breast cancer is thought to be the most curable form of the three major subtypes because it responds well to hormone therapy and has the propensity to spread slowly.

3. Triple-negative breast cancer

Most breast cancers that lack one of the aforementioned molecular receptors fall under the category of triple-negative breast cancer, also known as basal breast cancer. Beyond this, there may not be much in common among triple-negative breast cancers.

Triple-negative breast cancer is the most challenging subtype to treat because there is no receptor in these cancers that, when targeted, significantly influences the illness. The outlook for this subtype is frequently worse than those for others because it also tends to be more aggressive.

The term "triple-negative" describes the absence of three distinct chemicals, or "receptors," made by breast cancer cells.

The body's particular proteins and hormones can communicate with or bind to the receptors on a cell. We refer to this as awareness. Numerous cellular processes are triggered by recognition.

At least one of the three receptors that promote the development and spread of the disease through recognition is present in the majority of breast cancers. These are estrogen and progesterone receptors as well as the HER2 protein.

These receptors are used by doctors to treat breast cancer with medications that prevent detection. None of the three receptors are present in TNBC. Drugs that target these receptors do not, therefore, have any effect on TNBC. Various medications must be used.

One of the most aggressive forms of breast cancer is triple-negative, which also has rapid growth and a high incidence of recurrence.

Spread of breast cancer

When cancer cells enter the blood or lymphatic system and are then transported to other parts of the body, breast cancer can spread.

Your body's immune system includes the lymph (or lymphatic) system. It is a network of organs, ducts, and lymph nodes that cooperate to gather and transport clear lymph fluid through the bodily tissues and into the blood. Lymph nodes are tiny, bean-sized glands. The clear lymph fluid inside the lymph veins contains tissue by-products and waste debris, as well as immune system cells.

Lymph arteries are utilized to drain lymph fluid from the breast. Cancer cells may infiltrate those lymphatic channels in the case of breast cancer and begin to proliferate in lymph nodes. The majority of breast lymphatic arteries empty into:

• Armpit lymph nodes (axillary lymph nodes)

• Lymph nodes located close to the breastbone in the chest (internal mammary lymph nodes)
• Around the collarbone, lymph nodes (supraclavicular [above the collar bone] and infraclavicular [below the collar bone] lymph nodes)
There is a greater likelihood that cancer cells will have metastasized (moved to other places in your body) if they have already migrated to your lymph nodes. Some women without cancer cells in their lymph nodes may eventually develop metastases, and not all women with cancer cells in their lymph nodes do so.

Chapter 2

Other breast cancer types

1. In situ ductal carcinoma

In a situation known as ductal carcinoma in situ (DCIS), cancer cells have developed in the milk ducts but have not yet migrated to adjacent tissue. The initial stage of ductal breast cancer is known as DCIS. It is sometimes referred to as breast cancer in its early stages.

DCIS can progress and infect neighboring tissue in certain patients. DCIS can remain inside the ducts for years in some people. Both cannot be distinguished from one another.

Radiation therapy, chemotherapy, or surgery are all options for treating DCIS.

2. inflammatory Breast cancer

An uncommon and aggressive kind of breast cancer is inflammatory breast cancer (IBC). The condition generally develops a swollen, red, and sore breast within a few days or weeks, instead of a lump.

No inflammation is to blame for these symptoms. Instead, cancer cells in the skin and soft tissue obstruct lymph veins, which is what causes them. The fluid known as lymph is clear and contains cells that assist the body fight infection and waste from the tissues. Vascular structures resembling veins carry it throughout the body. Lymph fills up in the breast, causing it to enlarge, when these channels are obstructed by cancer cells.

HER2-positive, hormone receptor-positive, and triple-negative are the three molecular subtypes of IBC that, like more prevalent types of breast cancer, can promote cancer's growth and spread. IBC is more frequently triple-negative or HER2-positive than non-inflammatory breast cancer. These subtypes affect a patient's prognosis and course of treatment.

IBC is a contagious illness with a 40% five-year survival rate, according to historical data. Yet, improvements in healthcare are enabling more individuals to live longer. According to recent research, patients with stage III IBC have a five-year survival percentage closer to 70%, and patients with stage IV IBC have a five-year survival rate as high as 50%.

3. Breast cancer in men

Thousands of men are diagnosed with breast cancer each year in the United States, even though the disease usually affects women.

Male breast cancer has a marginally lower five-year survival rate than female breast cancer. The reduced survival rate has a lot of distinct causes. One is the patient's advanced age and the associated health risks. The average age of a male breast cancer patient at the time of diagnosis is 67, compared to 62 for females.

Also, when male breast cancer is discovered, it is often further along. Both the tumor and the likelihood that cancer has spread to nearby lymph nodes tend to be larger. Doctors blame a general lack of knowledge about male breast cancer as well as the absence of comprehensive screening for the condition for these later diagnoses.

Male breast cancer types

Similar to female breast cancer, the molecular receptor status of the cancer cells can be used to categorize male breast cancer.

On the surface of cancer cells are chemicals called receptors. Some proteins and hormones in the body of the patient can either bond with them or be recognized by them. Researchers have discovered receptors that, when bound to a certain protein or hormone, promote the growth of breast cancer cells. Cancer medications can reduce or stop the progression of the disease by severing this link.
The three primary breast cancer receptor types (in both men and women) are:
• HER2-positive, a protein that encourages cell division and development. Cancers that are HER2-positive have considerably higher than average levels of the HER2 protein.
• Possessing hormone receptors, which identify progesterone and estrogen.
• Triple-negative, which does not recognize progesterone, estrogen, or HER2. This breast cancer subtype is the hardest to treat because there is no molecular receptor to block.
Around 90% of male breast cancers are HER2-positive, while 9% of them are also hormone receptor-positive.

Male risk factors for breast cancer

A risk factor is something that makes someone more likely to get cancer. Several risk factors for male breast cancer have been recognized by medical professionals.

• BRCA variations The BRCA1 and BRCA2 genes function normally to prevent the growth of cancers. A mutant BRCA gene increases the risk of developing breast cancer in a person. In contrast to 5%–10% of female breast cancer patients, about 8%–15% of male breast cancer patients had a BRCA mutation. BRCA mutations are associated with ovarian, pancreatic, and melanoma cancers in addition to breast cancer.

• Breast cancer in the family: Men who have a parent, sibling, or child who has the disease are twice as likely to develop the disease themselves.

• Age: Men have a higher risk of developing breast cancer as they get older.

• Obesity

• Gynecomastia, or swollen breasts brought on by an imbalance in hormones or particular drugs

• Radiation exposure, frequently in connection with the treatment of another malignancy

• Race: Non-Hispanic white men have a lower risk of male breast cancer than African-American men do.

Symptoms of male breast cancer

The signs and symptoms of male breast cancer are remarkably similar to those of female breast cancer. They consist of:

• A breast lump or bulk
• Bulge or lump under the arm
• Changes to the breast skin, such as skin redness and thickness that gives the skin an orange-peel feel
• Dimpling or puckering on the breast
• Discharge from the nipple
• Scaliness on the nipple, which can occasionally extend to the areola
• The nipple's ability to change direction, pull to one side, or turn inside.
• An ulcer that sometimes extends to the areola of the breast or nipple
• Increased breast enlargement

4. A metaplastic breast cancer

It is uncommon and aggressive to have metaplastic breast cancer. A rapidly expanding tumor or lump in the breast is typically how it is found.

Breast cancer that originated in a milk duct and has expanded to surrounding tissue outside the duct is known as invasive ductal carcinoma. The tumor frequently resembles this malignancy during imaging studies. Yet, metaplastic breast cancer tumors are typically larger when they are discovered.

Metaplastic breast cancer cells resemble a variety of cancer kinds when viewed under a microscope. This once led medical professionals to think that it initially begins as two distinct tumors that eventually merge. Emerging evidence, however, points to metaplastic breast cancer as a single malignancy that may have started in very young cells with the capacity to differentiate into many types of mature cells.

The prognosis for metaplastic breast cancer

Metaplastic breast cancer grows more quickly than other types of breast cancer and is more likely to metastasize or spread to other regions of the body.

However, after successful initial treatment, it is more likely to return.
Patients with metaplastic breast cancer have a five-year survival rate of about 55%. The current survival rate may be higher because those who were diagnosed within the last few years and may have received newer, more potent therapies are not included in this statistic.

Treatment for metaplastic breast cancer

Less than 1% of all breast cancer diagnoses are for metaplastic breast cancer. Due of the condition's rarity, there have been relatively few clinical trials specifically devoted to it. According to current recommendations, it should be treated similarly to other breast tumors of the same stage and characteristics.
Triple-negative receptor status is present in the majority of metaplastic breast tumors. The estrogen receptor, progesterone receptor, and HER2 gene/protein are not overexpressed in these breast tumors. Triple-negative tumors are difficult to treat

using medications that target these characteristics of cancer cells. There is a need for further treatment plans.

Treatment normally begins with chemotherapy to decrease the tumor if the patient's cancer is discovered before it has progressed past the breast and nearby lymph nodes. Immunotherapy may also be used in this situation. Following this course of treatment, surgery and perhaps radiation therapy are used.

Chemotherapy or other cancer medications, either by themselves or in combination, are typically used to treat cancer that has spread past the breast and the lymph nodes nearby. Radiation may be used to lessen the discomfort brought on by a tumor mass.

5. Breast cancer that has spread

There is no specific type of advanced breast cancer, commonly known as metastatic breast cancer and stage IV breast cancer. It is instead any breast cancer that has progressed to the bones, brain, liver, or lungs in addition to the breast and adjacent lymph nodes. Although the condition may affect other organs, it is nonetheless treated and thought of as breast cancer.

The majority of advanced breast cancer cases are not thought to be treatable. Instead, they are handled like a persistent disease. The purpose of care is to

extend the life and preserve the patient's standard of living. Many metastatic breast cancer patients can enjoy long, healthy lives because of new medications and treatments.

6. Breast Paget disease

According to the National Cancer Institute, Paget disease is an uncommon type of breast cancer that accounts for 1-4% of all breast cancer cases. The areola is frequently affected after the nipple, where the illness first manifests. Numerous patients with Paget disease may also have a tumor or tumors in the breast that is impacted.

Paget disease of the breast is characterized by the following symptoms:

• Eczema-like skin changes on the nipple and/or areola, including crusting, thickness, and flakiness of the skin

• Nipple or areola tingling or burning

• An ulcer on the nipple or areola;

• A lump or lumps in the breast next to the affected nipple

• An inverted or flattened nipple
• A discharge from the nipple that is yellow or red.
Several of these symptoms can be misdiagnosed as
eczema or dermatitis, two skin disorders. As a result,

before Paget illness is identified, many people
exhibit symptoms for several months. The Paget
disease survival rate is marginally lower than the
general survival rate for breast cancer, in part
because of these later-than-usual diagnoses. The
likelihood of a cure is high if the illness is
discovered early, though.
The breast should be scanned if a doctor suspects a
patient has Paget disease of the breast. An
ultrasound or a mammogram may be used to do this.
A small sample of the tissue is taken if anything
abnormal is visible in the picture, such as a mass or
calcified tissue. This frequently happens during the
imaging test. A pathologist will then examine the
tissue sample to determine a diagnosis.
Yet, the patient might still have cancer if the biopsy
and pictures are clear. At this stage, a direct biopsy
of the nipple and/or areola is required.
Breast Paget disease is treated similarly to other
forms of breast cancer. The major distinction
happens during surgery. The nipple and areola must

be removed when a patient has surgery for Paget disease, whether it's a lumpectomy or a mastectomy.

Causes and Risk Factors for Breast Cancer

Although the exact cause of breast cancer is unknown, some factors increase your risk of developing it. Age, genetics, past medical history, and diet are all important. some are under your control; you can't with others.

Risk Factors for Breast Cancer You Can't Control

• **Age**. Women over 50 are more likely than younger women to develop breast cancer.
• **Race:** Before menopause, breast cancer is more common in African American women than in white women.

• **Dense breasts.** It could be challenging to detect malignancies on mammography if your breasts have more connective tissue than fatty tissue.

• **A personal cancer history.** If you have certain benign breast conditions, your probabilities are

somewhat increased. If you've already battled breast cancer, they rise more dramatically.

• **Ancestral history.** You are two times more likely to develop the condition if a first-degree female relative (mother, sister, or daughter) did. Your risk is at least tripled if you have two or more first-degree relatives who have had the disease. This is particularly true if they developed cancer before menopause or if both breasts were afflicted. If your father or brother has breast cancer, the chances may also increase.

• **Genes.** Some occurrences of familial breast cancer are caused by mutations in the BRCA1 and BRCA2 genes. One in 200 women carries one of these genes. They increase your risk of developing cancer but do not guarantee it. You have a 7 in 10 probability of developing breast cancer by the time you are 80 if you have a BRCA1 or BRCA2 mutation. These genes are associated with pancreatic cancer, and male breast cancer, and they increase your risk of developing ovarian cancer as well. The PTEN gene, the ATM gene, the TP53 gene, the CHEK2 gene, the CDH1 gene, the STK11 gene, and the PALB2 gene are among the other gene alterations associated with an increased risk of developing breast cancer.

Compared to the BRCA genes, these genes have a lower risk of developing breast cancer.
• **Past menstrual cycles.** Your risk of breast cancer increases if:
o Your period begins before the age of 12.
o Your periods continue until you are 55 years old.
• **Radiation.** Before the age of 40, you underwent treatment for tumors including Hodgkin's lymphoma, which increases your risk of developing breast cancer.
• **Diethylstilbene (DES).** Between 1940 and 1971, doctors prescribed this medication to stop miscarriages. Your risk of developing breast cancer rises if you or your mother took it.

The Risk Factors For Breast Cancer You Can Control

• **Physical exercise.** Your odds are better the less you move.

• **Diet and weight.** After menopause, being overweight increases your risk.
• **Alcohol.** Breast cancer risk is increased by regular drinking, especially more than one drink each day.
• **Previous sexual activity.**
o Your first child is born after you are 30.

o You don't nurse your baby.
o Your pregnancy is not at full term.
• **Hormone therapy.** Your likelihood can increase if you:
o Use estrogen and progesterone-containing hormone replacement treatment for longer than five years while going through menopause. Five years after you stop receiving treatment, this increase in breast cancer risk returns to normal.
o Employ certain hormonal birth control techniques, such as hormone-containing pills, injections, implants, IUDs, skin patches, or vaginal rings. Nonetheless, the majority of women with a high risk of developing breast cancer do not. On the other hand, there are no identified risk factors in 75% of women who acquire breast cancer.

Chapter 3

Diagnose and Testing

The majority of breast cancer types can be quickly identified through microscopic examination of a biopsy sample taken from the breast's afflicted area. Moreover, some forms of breast cancer necessitate specialist lab tests.

Mammography and physical examination of the breasts by a healthcare professional can both provide an approximate possibility that a lump is cancerous and may also pick up on other abnormalities, such as a straightforward cyst. When these tests are unhelpful, a medical professional may take a sample of the lump's fluid for microscopic inspection (a process called fine needle aspiration, or fine needle aspiration and cytology, or FNAC) to help make a diagnosis. It is possible to perform a needle aspiration in a medical office or clinic. If the lump is not under the skin, a local anesthetic may not be required to numb the breast tissue to prevent pain during the treatment. Clear fluid from a bulge is

nearly impossible to be carcinogenic, but bloody fluid can be examined under a microscope to look for malignant cells. Breast cancer can be accurately diagnosed with FNAC, mammography, and physical examination of the breasts altogether.
Additional biopsy alternatives include excisional biopsy, which involves removing the entire lump, core biopsy, which involves removing a part of the breast mass, and vacuum-assisted breast biopsy. The results of a physical examination by a healthcare professional, a mammogram, and any additional tests that might be carried out under unique conditions (such as imaging by ultrasound or MRI) are frequently sufficient to support excisional biopsy as the primary diagnostic and therapeutic approach.

Classification

There are various grading systems used to categorize breast cancers. Each of them affects the prognosis and may change how a patient responds to treatment. All of these elements are best included in a description of breast cancer.

1. Histopathology. Typically, breast cancer is categorized mostly based on histological appearance. The majority of breast cancers are classed as ductal or lobular carcinomas because they develop from the epithelium lining the ducts or lobules. The term "carcinoma in situ" refers to the development of low-grade malignant or precancerous cells within a specific tissue compartment, such as the mammary duct, without the surrounding tissue being invaded. In contrast, the original tissue compartment is not the only place where invasive cancer can spread.

2. Grade. Grading compares the breast cancer cells' appearance to that of healthy breast tissue. In an organ like the breast, normal cells differentiate or take on particular shapes and forms that represent

their role as a component of that organ. Cells that are cancerous stop differentiating. The milk ducts' normally structured cell linings, which line up in a logical pattern, become jumbled in malignancy. Uncontrollable cell division happens. Uniformity decreases in cell nuclei. The degree of differentiation of the cells is categorized by pathologists as well differentiated (low grade), moderately differentiated (intermediate grade), and poorly differentiated (high grade), depending on how much of the characteristics of normal breast cells they still retain. A worse prognosis can be expected from tumors that have poor differentiation (their tissue is least similar to normal breast tissue).

3. Stage. The size of the tumor (T), whether or not the tumor has progressed to the armpit lymph nodes (N), and whether or not the tumor has metastasized (M) are the three factors used in the TNM staging of breast cancer (i.e. spread to a more distant part of the body). A worse prognosis is associated with bigger size, nodal dissemination, and metastasis. Here are the key phases:

• Stage 0 refers to either ductal carcinoma in situ (DCIS) or lobular carcinoma in situ, which are precancerous or marker conditions (LCIS).

• Stages 1-3 are found in local or breast lymph nodes.

• Stage 4 cancer, often known as "metastatic" cancer, has progressed beyond the breast and local lymph nodes and has a worse prognosis.

In certain circumstances, imaging examinations may be used to help stage the patient and check for indicators of metastatic cancer. The dangers of PET scans, CT scans, and bone scans, which subject the patient to a significant dose of potentially hazardous ionizing radiation, outweigh any potential advantages in patients with breast cancer with minimal risk of spreading.

4. Status of receptors. Receptors are present in the cytoplasm, nucleus, and surface of breast cancer cells. Hormones and other chemical messengers bind to receptors, changing the cell as a result. Estrogen receptor (ER), progesterone receptor (PR), and HER2 are three crucial receptors that breast cancer cells may or may not possess.

Because ER+ cancer cells (i.e., cancer cells with estrogen receptors) rely on estrogen to develop, they can be treated with medications that block the effects of estrogen (such as tamoxifen) and typically have a better prognosis. HER2+ breast cancers tend

to be more aggressive than HER2- breast cancers when left untreated, but HER2+ cancer cells react to medications such as the monoclonal antibody trastuzumab (in combination with traditional chemotherapy), which has considerably improved the prognosis. Triple-negative cells express receptors for other hormones, such as the androgen receptor and prolactin receptor, but lack any of these three receptor types (estrogen receptors, progesterone receptors, or HER2).

5. DNA tests. Breast cancer cells and normal cells have been compared using DNA testing of many kinds, including DNA microarrays. Selecting the most suitable treatment for a certain DNA type may be aided by the unique changes in a given breast cancer, which can be used to identify the disease in several ways.

Stages of Breast Cancer

• **Breast cancer that is noninvasive, early stage, or stage 0.** There are no indications that the disease has progressed to the lymph nodes; it exclusively affects the breast (your doctor will call this carcinoma in situ).

• **Breast cancer in Stage I.** The malignancy has not spread and is no larger than 2 cm.

• **Breast cancer in Stage IIA.** The tumor is o Less than 2 cm in diameter; underarm lymph nodes are affected.

o More than 2 but smaller than 5 cm in diameter; lymph nodes unaffected.

• **Breast cancer at Stage IIB.** a tumor that is

o More than 5 cm in diameter and not involving the underarm lymph nodes

o Lymph nodes involved, larger than 2 but less than 5 centimeters wide.

• Breast cancer in stage IIIA or locally advanced breast cancer:

o A tumor that is over 5 cm in size and has metastasized to the lymph nodes beneath the arm or close to the breastbone.

o Any size tumor with adherent malignant lymph nodes or surrounding tissue.

• Breast cancer in Stage IIIB. any tumor, regardless of size, that has migrated to the chest wall or skin.

• Breast cancer at stage IIIC. Any size tumor that has engulfed more lymph nodes and spread farther.

• Breast cancer in Stage IV (metastatic). is a tumor of any size that has metastasized outside of the breast, such as to the bones, lungs, liver, brain, or distant lymph nodes.

Screening

Breast cancer screening is the process of checking the status of otherwise healthy women for the disease to make an earlier diagnosis with the hope of improving outcomes. Mammography, genetic testing, ultrasound, and magnetic resonance imaging are just a few of the screening tests that have been used.

Feeling the breast for lumps or other abnormalities is part of a clinical or self-breast exam. While self-breast exams are carried out by the individual, clinical breast exams are performed by medical professionals. Both types of breast exams are not effective, according to the evidence, as by the time a lump is big enough to be identified, it has probably been developing for a while and will soon be big enough to be found without an exam. X-rays are used in mammographic screening for breast cancer to look for any lumps or masses that are not normal. A technician compresses the breast during a screening while taking many images from various angles. Whereas diagnostic mammography concentrates on a particular lump or area of concern, a general mammogram takes pictures of the entire breast.

Several national organizations advise breast cancer screening. The U.S. Preventive Services Task Force and American College of Physicians recommend mammography every two years in women between the ages of 50 and 74, the Council of Europe recommends mammography between the ages of 50 and 69 with the majority of programs using a 2-year frequency, the European Commission recommends

mammography from the ages of 45 to 75 every 2 to 3 years, and in Canada screening is advised between the ages of 50 and 74 at a frequency of 2 to 3 years. The American Cancer Society also recommends that women get mammograms every year starting at age 40. These task force studies note that a tiny but considerable rise in radiation-induced breast cancer is one of the dangers of more frequent mammograms, in addition to unneeded surgery and anxiety.

According to the Cochrane collaboration (2013), the highest quality data does not show a decrease in cancer-specific or overall cause-specific mortality as a result of screening mammography. When less rigorous trials are included in the analysis, there is a 0.05% drop in mortality from breast cancer (1 fewer death per 2000 over 10 years, or a 15% relative decrease from breast cancer). Overdiagnosis and overtreatment rates rise by 30% as a result of screening over ten years (3 to 14 per 1000), and more than half of patients will have at least one false-positive test. As a result, it is unclear whether mammography screenings are more beneficial or harmful. According to Cochrane, "it consequently seems no longer helpful to visit for breast cancer

screening" at any age because of recent advancements in breast cancer treatment and the dangers of false positives from breast cancer screening leading to unneeded treatment. It is unknown whether using MRI as a screening tool has more risks or benefits compared to using traditional mammography.

Prevention

Lifestyle

By keeping a healthy weight, cutting back on alcohol usage, upping physical exercise, and breastfeeding, women can lower their risk of breast cancer. In the US, 42% in the UK, 28% in Brazil, and 20% in China, these changes may be able to prevent 38% of breast cancer cases. All age groups, including postmenopausal women, benefit from a moderate activity like brisk walking. High levels of physical activity cut breast cancer risk by 14% on average. Obesity reduction and regular physical activity promotion strategies may also lower the risk of diabetes and cardiovascular disease, among other health advantages. Strong evidence that higher levels of physical activity and less sedentary time are likely to reduce the risk of breast cancer, with results largely consistent across breast cancer subtypes, was identified in a study that included information from 130,957 women of European ancestry.

2016 saw recommendations from the American Cancer Society and the American Society of Clinical Oncology that patients should consume a diet rich in fruits, vegetables, whole grains, and legumes. Breast cancer risk is 10% lower in people who consume a lot of citrus fruit. Omega-3 polyunsaturated fatty acids from marine sources seem to lessen the risk. A high intake of foods containing soy may lower the risk.

Emergency surgery

Women with BRCA1 and BRCA2 mutations, which are linked to a significantly increased risk for an eventual diagnosis of breast cancer, may be considered for removal of both breasts before any cancer has been diagnosed or any suspicious lump or other lesion has appeared (a procedure known as "prophylactic bilateral mastectomy" or "risk-reducing mastectomy"). Only women who pose the greatest risk should undergo this treatment, according to the available evidence. After genetic counseling, BRCA testing is advised for people with a high family risk. It is not typically advised. This is due to the wide variety of changes that can occur in the BRCA genes, from benign polymorphisms to blatantly harmful frameshift mutations. Most of the observable alterations in genes have unknown effects. Testing on an individual with average risk will likely produce one of these ambiguous, pointless results. The contralateral risk-reducing mastectomy (CRRM), which involves removing the second breast in a breast cancer patient, may lower the risk of developing cancer in the second breast, although it is not known whether doing so increases survival. Women who test positive for defective BRCA1 or BRCA2 genes increasingly elect to undergo risk-reducing surgery. In addition, the typical waiting period for the treatment is two years, which is far longer than is advised.

Medications

The particular estrogen receptor modulators raise the risk of thrombosis and endometrial cancer while decreasing the risk of breast cancer. The danger of death has not changed at all. As a result, they are not advised for the control of breast cancer in women at ordinary risk, but they should be provided to those at high risk who are over 35. After finishing a treatment regimen with these drugs, the benefit of decreased breast cancer continues for no less than

five more years. Exemestane and anastrozole are
two examples of aromatase inhibitors that would be
more effective than tamoxifen at lowering the risk of
breast cancer without increasing the possibility of
endometrial cancer or thrombosis.

Chapter 4

Breast Cancer Therapy and Management

The stage of cancer and the patient's age are two variables that affect how breast cancer is managed. When cancer is more advanced or there is a higher risk of cancer recurrence after therapy, treatments are more aggressive.

Surgery is the traditional first step in the treatment of breast cancer, which may then be followed by radiation therapy, chemotherapy, or both. A multidisciplinary approach should be used whenever possible. Hormone-blocking therapy is frequently used over several years to treat tumors that have hormone receptors. Although this area of treatment is still under investigation, monoclonal antibodies or other immune-modulating therapies may be used in some cases with metastatic and other advanced stages of breast cancer.

Surgery

During surgery, the tumor is physically removed, frequently along with some of the surrounding tissue. During the procedure, one or more lymph nodes may be biopsied; increasingly, a sentinel lymph node biopsy is used to sample the lymph nodes.

The following procedures are common:

• Mastectomy: Whole breast removal.

• Quadrantectomy: A quarter of the breast is removed.

• Removal of a little portion of the breast during a lumpectomy.

Breast reconstruction surgery, a type of plastic surgery, can be done to enhance the treated site's cosmetic appeal after the tumor has been removed, if the patient so chooses. Women can also choose to have a flat chest or use breast prostheses to mimic breast undergarments. Using a nipple prosthetic is possible at any point after a mastectomy.

Medication

Adjuvant therapy refers to medications taken both before and after surgery. Neoadjuvant therapy refers to treatments given before surgery, such as chemotherapy. When combined with other treatments, aspirin may lower breast cancer-related mortality.

Hormone-blocking medicines, chemotherapy, and monoclonal antibodies are the three primary categories of drugs now used for adjuvant breast cancer treatment.

Hormonal treatment

For some breast tumors to keep developing, estrogen is necessary. They are distinguishable because they have progesterone receptors (PR+) and estrogen receptors (ER+) on their surface (sometimes referred to together as hormone receptors). These ER+ tumors can be treated with either medication that blocks the receptors, like tamoxifen, or drugs that use an aromatase inhibitor, like anastrozole or letrozole, to prevent the generation of estrogen. Tamoxifen usage is advised for ten years. [157] Tamoxifen increases the risk of postmenopausal bleeding, endometrial hyperplasia, polyps, and endometrial cancer. Combining tamoxifen with an intrauterine system that releases levonorgestrel may result in an increase in vaginal bleeding after one to two years, but it also somewhat reduces endometrial hyperplasia and polyps, though not necessarily endometrial cancer. It is advised to take letrozole for five years.

Only women who have experienced menopause should use aromatase inhibitors, but in this group, they appear to be superior to tamoxifen. Because the active aromatase in postmenopausal women differs from the dominant version in premenopausal women, these medicines are unable to block the premenopausal women's predominant aromatase. Intact ovarian function in premenopausal women should prevent them from taking aromatase inhibitors (unless they are also on treatment to stop their ovaries from working). Endocrine or aromatase therapy can be used in conjunction with CDK inhibitors.

Chemotherapy

Chemotherapy is typically used for breast cancer cases in stages 2-4 and is especially helpful in ER-negative (ER-) illnesses. Combinations of chemotherapeutic drugs are given, often for intervals of three to six months. One of the most used regimens, called "AC," combines doxorubicin and cyclophosphamide. When a taxane medicine, like docetaxel, is added, the treatment is referred to as "CAT." Cyclophosphamide, methotrexate, and fluorouracil are other typical treatments (or "CMF"). The majority of chemotherapy drugs function by killing rapidly expanding and/or rapidly replicating cancer cells, either by inflicting DNA damage during replication or through other means. The drugs also harm rapidly proliferating normal cells, which could have negative side effects. For instance, the most dangerous side effect of doxorubicin is damage to the heart muscle.

Monoclonal antibodies

The five-year disease-free survival of stage 1-3 HER2-positive breast tumors with trastuzumab, a monoclonal antibody to HER2, has increased to about 87% (overall survival of 95%). The HER2 gene or its protein product is overexpressed in 25% to 30% of breast cancers, and HER2 overexpression in breast cancer is linked to a higher risk of disease recurrence and a worse prognosis. However, trastuzumab is exceedingly expensive, and using it may result in major adverse effects (around 2% of patients acquire significant heart damage). In cases of severe disease, the antibody pertuzumab is also advised in addition to trastuzumab and chemotherapy since it suppresses HER2 dimerization.

Breast cancer medication therapy with specific targets

Certain medications can specifically target cancer-causing cell traits. If your breast cancer has spread to other parts of your body, your doctor may advise you to take targeted medication therapy. Some of the most well-liked treatments for breast cancer include monoclonal antibodies (such trastuzumab, pertuzumab, as well as margetuximab), antibody-drug conjugates (like ado-trastuzumab emtansine as well as fam-trastuzumab deruxtecan), or even kinase inhibitors (such as lapatinib, neratinib, and tucatinib)

Radiation

Following surgery, radiotherapy is administered to the area of the tumor bed and local lymph nodes to eradicate any tiny tumor cells that may have evaded the surgical procedure. The tumor microenvironment may benefit when it is treated with targeted intraoperative radiation during surgery. Brachytherapy or external beam radiotherapy are two ways that radiation therapy can be administered (internal radiotherapy). Traditionally, radiation for breast cancer is administered following surgery. Furthermore, radiation can be administered during breast cancer surgery. When breast cancer is treated by removing only the lump, radiation is thought to be crucial since it can reduce the risk of recurrence by 50–66% (half–2/3 reduction of risk) (Lumpectomy or Wide local excision). Partial breast irradiation does not provide the same cancer control in the breast as treating the entire breast and may have harsher side effects in cases of early breast cancer.

Supplied care

Treatment after primary breast cancer treatment, sometimes known as "follow-up care," can be rigorous and involve routine laboratory tests on asymptomatic people to detect potential metastases early. According to a review, follow-up programs that only include annual mammograms and routine physical exams are just as successful as more comprehensive ones when it comes to recurrence early detection, overall survival, and quality of life.

Multidisciplinary rehabilitation programs, which frequently include exercise, education, and psychological support, may short-term increase social involvement, psychosocial adjustment, and functional abilities in breast cancer patients.

After radiotherapy or breast cancer surgery, upper limb issues like shoulder and arm pain, weakness, and restricted movement are frequently seen as side effects. An exercise regimen that is started 7–10 days following surgery helps lessen upper limb issues, according to UK studies.

Prognosis Predictive variables

Breast cancer stage-specific prognosis Stage 5-year survival

100% at Stage I

90% Stage II

70% Stage III

30% Stage IV

Traditional classification systems of breast cancer place the most emphasis on the stage of the disease since it has a bigger impact on the prognosis than any other factor. Size, local involvement, lymph node status, and the presence of metastatic disease are all factors in staging. The prognosis becomes worse the later the diagnosis is made. The aggressiveness of the cancer cells and the extent of the disease's invasion into the lymph nodes, chest wall, skin, or elsewhere raise the stage. The existence of cancer-free areas and nearly normal cell behavior lowers the stage (grading). Until the cancer is aggressive, size has little bearing on staging. For instance, ductal carcinoma in situ (DCIS) that affects the entire breast will still be in stage zero and have a very good outlook.

• Cancers at stage 1 (including DCIS and LCIS) have a very good prognosis and are typically treated with a lumpectomy and occasionally radiotherapy.

• Surgery (lumpectomy or mastectomy with or without lymph node removal), chemotherapy (with trastuzumab for HER2+ tumors), and occasionally radiation are typically used to treat stage 2 and stage 3 malignancies, which have a progressively worse prognosis and a higher chance of recurrence (particularly following large cancers, multiple positive nodes or lumpectomy).

• Cancer that has spread to distant areas, or stage 4, has a dismal prognosis and is treated with a variety of surgical, radiation, chemotherapeutic, and targeted therapies.

By contrasting breast cancer cells with healthy breast cells, the grade of breast cancer is determined. The prognosis is better and the cancer cells develop more slowly the closer they are to normal cells. When cells lack proper differentiation, they exhibit immaturity, divide quickly, and have the propensity to spread. A grade of 1 is awarded for well-differentiated work, a grade of 2 for moderately differentiated work, and a higher grade of 3 or 4 for poorly or undifferentiated work (depending upon the scale used). The Nottingham scheme is the most popular grading system.

Due to several variables, post-menopausal women tend to have a worse prognosis than younger women under the age of 40 or older women over the age of 80. They might be breastfeeding infants, their breasts might alter with their menstrual cycles, and they might not even be aware of the changes. Hence, when diagnosed, younger women are typically in a more advanced stage. The greater risk of disease recurrence in younger breast cancer patients may be due to biological variables.

Psychological considerations

Not every breast cancer patient has the same experience with their condition. Age, among other things, can significantly affect how someone responds to receiving a breast cancer diagnosis. Several chemotherapy regimens used to treat breast cancer, especially those that use hormones to suppress ovarian function, cause early menopause in

premenopausal women with estrogen-receptor-
positive breast cancer.

Psychological therapies, such as cognitive
behavioral therapy, can improve symptoms
including anxiety, depression, and mood disruption
in women with non-metastatic breast cancer. During
adjuvant therapy, physical activity programs may
also have positive benefits on the health-related
quality of life, anxiety, fitness, and physical activity
in breast cancer patients.

Cancer type-specific prognosis

The classification of DCIS into comedo (i.e.,
cribriform, micropapillary, and solid) and non
comedo subtypes offers further prognostic data on
the chance of progression or local recurrence. In
general, comedo DCIS has a worse prognosis than
non comedo DCIS (see Histology).

Within 15 years after their LCIS diagnosis, 10–20%
of women with LCIS will develop invasive breast
cancer. LCIS is therefore regarded as an indicator of
elevated breast cancer risk.

The most often found breast tumor, infiltrating
ductal carcinoma, often spreads through lymphatic
channels. Infiltrating lobular carcinoma often

spreads to the axillary lymph nodes first, similar to ductal cancer. It also has the propensity to be more multifocal, though. Nonetheless, it has a prognosis that is similar to ductal carcinoma.

Despite the poor prognostic characteristics connected with this form of breast cancer, such as ER-negative, high tumor grade, and high proliferative rates, typical or classic medullary carcinomas frequently have a fair prognosis. The overall survival and prognosis, however, are not as good as previously reported, according to an examination of 609 medullary breast cancer specimens from various stage I and II NSABP (National Surgical Adjuvant Breast as well as Bowel Project) guidelines. Moreover, the prognosis is worse for atypical medullary carcinomas.

Overall, the prognosis for individuals with mucinous carcinoma is very good, with a 10-year survival rate of greater than 80%. Similar to this, tubular carcinoma has a very good probability of overall survival and a low frequency of lymph node involvement. These patients frequently just require local radiation therapy and breast-conserving surgery due to the good prognosis.

Low mitotic activity in cystic papillary carcinoma leads to a more indolent course and a favorable prognosis. Although over 70% of cases are ER-positive, invasive micropapillary ductal carcinoma has a more aggressive character. Invasive micropapillary ductal carcinoma was found in 83 cases (6%) out of 1400 cases of invasive carcinoma, according to a retrospective analysis.

Moreover, this subtype is prone to lymph node metastasis (incidence, 70–90%), and the quantity of lymph nodes affected seems to be related to survival.

Even after adjusting for stage, most published case series for metaplastic breast cancer show a worse prognosis than for infiltrating ductal carcinoma, with a 3-year overall survival rate of 48-71% and 15-60%, respectively, for 3-year disease-free survival. Large tumor size and later stages have become predictors of poor survival rates and prognosis in the majority of case series. It does not seem that nodal status affects mortality in metaplastic breast cancer. In 75% of instances, Paget disease of the breast is linked to underlying breast cancer. Satisfactory outcomes are possible with breast-conserving surgery, however, this comes with a chance of local recurrence. A palpable breast tumor, lymph node involvement, a particular histologic type, and young age are all indicators of a poor prognosis. There is typically an invasive component to Paget disease when there is a palpable mass, and the 5-year survival rate is lower (20–60%). A better 5-year survival rate (75-100%) is seen in patients without an underlying palpable mass.

A cardiovascular condition

Women with breast cancer have an elevated risk of cardiovascular disease (CVD). The cardiotoxic side effects of several breast cancer medications are a contributing factor in the increase (eg, chemotherapy, radiotherapy, and targeted therapy such as trastuzumab). In addition, there are various risk factors for both CVD and breast cancer, such as smoking, being overweight, and eating a normal Western diet.

Obesity and dyslipidemia are CVD risk factors that are more likely to occur in older breast cancer survivors than tumor recurrence. Breast cancer survivors have a higher risk of dying from a CVD in the population of older postmenopausal women than do women without a history of breast cancer. Seven years after a breast cancer diagnosis, the increased risk starts to show.

Chapter 5

Natural treatments for breast cancer

The following are some typical herbs that are used to treat breast cancer:

1. Echinacea

Echinacea is a member of the Asteraceae family. It is an untamed aromatic plant that is primarily grown in North America's Great Plains and eastern regions, while it is also made in Europe. The three Echinacea species—Echinacea purpurea, Echinacea angustifolia, and Echinacea pallida—are the most often encountered forms for use in herbal medicines. Nonetheless, E. purpurea is most frequently utilized in research and medical therapy. Purple coneflower, Kansas snakeroot, and black Sampson are a few popular names associated with echinacea. According to research, E. purpurea causes the investigating mice's natural killer cell count to increase. E.

purpurea may one day be used as a cancer treatment therapy (Steffani, 2005).

Flavonoids, which are found in echinacea, stimulate the immune system. Winston et al. provided support for this, and flavonoids encourage lymphocyte activity, which boosts macrophage phagocytosis, the activity of natural killer cells, and the induction of interferon assembly. They help minimize the negative effects of radiotherapy and chemotherapy.

2. Garlic

For hundreds of years, people have utilized garlic (Allium sativum) to treat a variety of diseases. There are a hundred or more therapeutically valuable secondary metabolites involved, such as alliin, alliinase, and allicin. Garlic oil contains alliin, an amino acid that when crushed into allicin becomes present. Allicin is one of the compounds that contain sulfur and is the source of the odor and medicinal effects of this substance. Ajoene, another molecule that holds sulfur, is present in garlic oil. Ajoene reduces the progression of cancer while selenium functions as an antioxidant. Garlic also contains bioflavonoids, cyanidin, and quercetin, which have antioxidant effects. Garlic's high concentration of organic sulfides and polysulfides is what gives it its anti-cancer properties. The lymphocytes and macrophages that are stimulated to produce anti-tumor activity do so by killing malignant cells and interfering with the metabolism of tumor cells. According to studies, garlic increases the amount of suppressor T cells and changes lymphocytes into a form that is poisonous to malignant cells. By changing the adhesion and attachment of malignant cells moving via the blood arteries, metastases are avoided. Ripe garlic extract boosts the body's immune system, speeds up the clearance of carcinogens from the body, and raises the activity of the detoxification enzyme all while preventing the harmful effects of carcinogens on DNA. According to research, the ripened garlic extract can also prevent the spread of many malignancies, including those of the colon, stomach, breast, lungs, and bladder. Garlic extract has the potential to reduce the side effects of chemotherapy and radiotherapy.

3. Curcumin

Turmeric's scientific name is Curcuma longa. Food is dyed a dark yellow with turmeric. The rhizome and rootstock of turmeric contain curcumin, the compound that gives it its color. Due to its phenolic components, curcumin is recognized to have anti-cancerous properties. Turmeric prevents the spread of stomach, lung, breast, and skin cancer (Winston, 1999)

Curcumin, an antioxidant, affects the formation of eicosanoids such as prostaglandin E-2 (PGE-2). It also has an anti-inflammatory effect on people. According to research, curcumin inhibits the initiation, promotion, and propagation stages of cancer growth. Turmeric prevents the development of nitrosamine, which increases the body's natural antioxidant defenses. Curcumin increases the levels of glutathione and other non-protein sulphydryls, which then directly affect several enzymes.

4. Burdock

Burdock's botanical name is Arctium lappa. Asia and Europe both have it and use it. Burdock is a medicinal plant that is used in numerous herbal treatments. Its root has a sweet flavor and gummy texture. Burdock was once helpful for treating arthritis, tonsillitis, and measles, however, these days it has been discovered that it has anticancer activity. It has several active components that affect how oncogenes change. Burdock has been used to treat cancers of the pancreas, ovary, bladder, malignant melanoma, and breast. It reduces the growth of the tumor, eases discomfort, and lengthens the period of survival. During cancer, a significant number of nutrients are needed to support the rapid proliferation and division of cells. Yet, cancer cells can survive under stressful conditions, such as low oxygen levels and low glucose levels, because these conditions are well tolerated by tumor cells. Arctigenin is an active component found in burdock seeds. Arctigenin has demonstrated the capacity to eradicate tumor cells with little nutrient input. Flavonoid and polyphenol anti-oxidants found in burdock root may have a suppressive effect on the growth of tumors. By using a root extract, healthy bodily cells are shielded from harmful substances, and cell mutation is reduced. Tannin, a phenolic molecule, is the most significant active component of burdock. It increases macrophage activity, inhibits the spread of malignancy, and maintains immune-modulatory capabilities (Potter, 1997).

5. Carotenoids

The green, leafy plant known as rose hips contains an active substance known as "carotenoids." Saffron, annatto, and paprika are just a few examples of the dyes made from these aromatic plants. Consuming fruits and vegetables has been associated with a reduction in the growth of several tumor types. Consuming carotenoids through food also reduces the risk of tumor development (Donaldson, 2004). The carotenoid compounds are strong antioxidants and exhibit a wide range of therapeutic properties, including the ability to hunt down free radicals, defend against oxidative cell damage, improve gap intersections, stimulate the immune system, and control the activity of enzymes that contribute to the development of cancer.

6. Green tea

The botanical name for green tea is Camellia sinensis. Polyphenolic chemicals are responsible for their anticancer action. A minor amount of polyphenol epigallocatechin (EGGG) is found in C. Sinensis. Green tea has been shown to have anticancer and antimutagenic properties by researchers. EGGG shields cells from DNA damage brought on by oxygen-reactive species (Lambert and Yang, 2003). According to studies done on animals, green tea polyphenols inhibit the division of cancer cells and promote the necrosis and death of tumor cells (Zaveri, 2006). Tea catechins stimulate the immune system, but they also prevent tumor cells from metastasizing and from forming new blood vessels. Green tea has been proven in certain trials to be protective against stomach and colon cancer. Tea and its principal catechins lower the risk of tumor development in several body organs. Green tea helps mitigate radiation's negative effects. The antioxidant activity of tea is the cause of all its positive effects.

7. Ginseng

Ginseng is known by the scientific name Panax ginseng. In China, Korea, Japan, and Russia, this perennial plant primarily flourishes. The dried root of this plant is a useful part. It can treat a variety of illnesses, including cancer. The active ingredients in ginseng have demonstrated that they diminish or stop the growth of tumor necrosis factor in mouse skin, stop the spread and metastasis of malignant cells, and increase the level of interferon. The components of ginseng may help prevent the development of other types of malignant cells. A Korean study that was also conducted concluded that ginseng lowers the risk of cancer in humans. The most potent and effective form of ginseng for reducing the risk of cancer is its extract and dried powder, as opposed to freshly sliced ginseng, its juice, or its tea. Ginseng keeps the tumor from developing by preventing the creation of DNA. The beneficial effects of P. ginseng's active ingredient include the restoration of natural killer cells damaged by chemotherapy and radiation therapy, as well as the induction of macrophages and improved antibody production.

8. Black cohosh

Black cohosh is officially known as Cimicifuga racemose. It is a shrub that can be found in North America's eastern woods. Black cohosh is most frequently utilized by breast cancer patients during radiotherapy and chemotherapy. Native Americans have used it for many years to treat dysmenorrhea, premenstrual discomfort, and menopausal symptoms. Moreover, it causes issues similar to abortion. a patented drug The primary ingredient in Lydia Pinkham's famed vegetable compound, which contained this herb. The pharmacopeia from the 19th century contained it as well. Drug stores offer a wide variety of black cohosh preparations.

Women who were advised by their doctor to stop using hormone replacement therapy (HRT) for women have done so. The majority of studies have demonstrated the herb's efficacy on menopausal symptoms. Although the active ingredients in black cohosh are unknown, triterpene glycosides are thought to be a key component. Trace amounts of resins, caffeic, ferulic, and fumarolic acids are also thought to be present. There are questions about the black cohosh's estrogenic and anti-estrogenic properties. Contradictory findings from many research investigations indicate that it either increases or decreases the formation of cancer cells in the culture. Black cohosh has synergistic effects for breast cancer patients when used in conjunction with other chemotherapy drugs, according to the research.

9. Flax seed

Flax seeds are tiny and hard-coated, and they are brown and golden. All the active ingredients are included in these tiny seeds. Omega 3 fatty acids, lignans, and dietary fiber are all abundant in flax seeds. Flax seeds contain estrogenic action as a result of the digestive tract's conversion of lignans to enterodiol and enterolactone. Flax seeds contain more strong phytoestrogens than soy products, and the use of flax seeds significantly alters the elimination of 2-hydoxyesterone compared to soy protein. It has been demonstrated by Lilian Thompson's research team at the University of

Toronto that powdered flax seeds contain potent anti-cancer properties. In a mouse experiment, cancer was first created by giving the mice carcinogens, and in one group, the anti-cancer properties of flax seed were discovered by adding lignin to the mice's diet. The tumor load has decreased as a result of this experiment. The malignancies were reduced with flax seeds and secoisolariciresinol glycoside.

10. Calcium

Skin contact with the sun produces vitamin D. In the summer, mere contact of the hands, arms, and face produces significant amounts of vitamin D. Simply standing in the sun on the beach until the skin turns pink is equivalent to taking 20,000 IU of vitamin D2 orally. Our bodies just need 1000 IU of vitamins per day to maintain a suitable level. In the absence of sunlight, the only way to maintain vitamin D levels is by oral intake. With other advantages, 4000 IU can be taken safely in a single day. The blood's active hormonal form of vitamin D is kept in check by the kidneys. This active form of vitamin D has anti-cancer properties. Vital organs of the body were able to function because of the ability to convert vitamin D's main circulating form, 25(OH) D, into the hormone form, 1, 25(OH) 2D. All of these organs have a local process that they use to change the circulating form into a hormonal form, and exposure to sunlight stimulates this mechanism.

Having Early-Stage Breast Cancer and Living Your Best Life

In recovering from early-stage breast cancer, taking care of your body and mind will improve your general health and give you the energy you need to battle. These are some methods you can use to position yourself for success.

• Watch Your Food and Drink

Your body is strengthened by healthy nutrients. Cancer patients only need to eat the same things as the rest of us, such as fruits and vegetables. There is no particular diet for cancer patients. Eat at least 2 1/2 cups of coffee per day. Use it with vegetables that are dark green, red, and orange.

whole grains. Seek 100% whole grain products including bread, cereal, and brown rice.

Fat. Choose foods with unsaturated fats like almonds, nut butter, avocados, and olive oil as your main sources.

Reduce your consumption of red and processed meat, sugar-sweetened beverages, processed meals, and alcohol.

Do not forget to drink adequate water. It's crucial if you struggle to keep meals down while receiving cancer therapy. Or if you've lost water due to diarrhea, a fever, or sweating. Try these alternatives if you find water to be too bland: herbal tea, fruit juice diluted in water, and fat-free soy milk

Make an effort to consume 8 to 10 glasses of liquid each day. Avoid drinking alcohol, black tea, and caffeinated cola as they can cause dehydration.

• Maintain Motion

According to research, staying active increases your chances of surviving longer after receiving a cancer diagnosis. However, you only need a modest quantity of exercise to experience the advantages, such as an increase in energy and mood as well as decreased tension and worry.

The following activities qualify as moderate exercise: gardening, walking, and dancing.

To increase your heart rate even further, try jogging, swimming, or playing tennis. Experts recommend 150 minutes of physical activity per week. just 30 minutes five days a week, each day. Strength training is another option, which you can do twice a week or more. Ask your doctor for advice on what is safe.

• Control fatigue

Most patients experience fatigue at some point during their treatment for breast cancer. Even after a restful night's sleep, you'll feel exhausted. Even after your therapy is over, you may still feel fatigued.

Keeping active is one way to combat weariness. Exercise might not even be on your mind right now. Yet, it might make you feel better. Start with 15 minutes of exercise and increase the duration gradually to an hour or more.

Obtain nutrition. Make sure you consume enough calories overall, protein, vitamins, and minerals. Consult a nutritionist or your doctor about any potential needs you may have.

Maintain a healthy sleep routine. Establish the practice of sleeping in and rising at a certain time each day. You can take brief naps. Simply aim to limit them to 30 minutes or less.

Make a daily plan. Ask for Help Save essential duties for when you're feeling your best and work little by little.

• Asking for assistance

whenever you need it is a crucial component of taking care of yourself once you have cancer.

Family and friends

Let your loved ones know how they can help by having a conversation with them. It can be a ride to the doctor, groceries, child care, or simply somebody to talk to.

Advisory services

Speaking with people who are going through cancer may also be beneficial. Support groups are a terrific place to share feelings and worries as well as get advice on how to manage cancer. Choose a group that most closely matches your needs. It can be one for those battling breast cancer or another type of cancer. Along with age- or sex-specific groups, other groups are treatment-focused.

Counseling

Consider speaking with a mental health expert if your daily life is being affected by feelings related to your cancer diagnosis. Their responsibility is to assist you in identifying the source of your worries and in learning how to manage the changes that cancer may cause. Your medical staff might be able to recommend someone who has experience working with cancer patients.

What Comes Next After a Breast Cancer Early Stage Diagnosis?

Everyone is affected differently by a cancer diagnosis. The news may require some time to sink in. At first, you could deny having a disease. Maybe you might experience intense despair, rage, or worry. But after you accept the diagnosis, you could also experience hope. These emotions are all normal.

You might be interested in what happens next as well. What you should know is as follows.

• **Read More.**

Become well-versed in the details of your particular cancer type. Consult your doctor What stage your disease is in?

Your breast or auxiliary lymph nodes, which are those near your armpit, are the only areas where early-stage breast cancer has not spread. The majority of Americans who are diagnosed with breast cancer are still in their early stages. What follows is included in that:

Stage 0 (ductal carcinoma in situ). Your milk ducts are affected by this type of malignancy.

Stages I–2. You have lymph nodes and breasts with tiny or large tumors.

Level IIIa. You could have more lymph nodes with cancer or larger tumors.

The type of treatment you'll require depends on the stage of your breast cancer. Radiation therapy and surgery are typically combined for patients. Before or after your surgery, you might undergo chemotherapy or take additional medications. Consult your physician to go over each treatment's adverse effects and recovery period. Before each appointment, make a list of your questions. Take a relative or pal with you, or make a note of what your doctor says. To comprehend everything on your own can be challenging.

• Engage Others

A diagnosis of cancer is a private matter. You decide to who you reveal yourself. Consider how much information you want to provide them. You want to inform the following persons about your sickness as soon as possible:

• Your partner or spouse; Your family; Your close pals; A Few Coworkers

You might need to inform your manager or a member of human resources that you are ill. If you need it, they'll assist you in figuring out how to take time off.

• Assemble your support group.

Cancer shouldn't be experienced alone. Moreover, social support can enhance the way you live before, during, and after therapy.

You might decide to rely on your partner or spouse. A trusted friend could end up being your rock. Or perhaps being around other cancer patients makes you feel more at ease. You can join support groups locally or nationally by asking your doctor about them.

You might also wish to expand your network by including the following people:

Develop a plan with your coworkers, social worker, therapist, and spiritual adviser.

You don't have to give up doing the activities you enjoy because of cancer. Moreover, if you can, try to maintain your normal routine. Discuss with your doctor how you might fit in treatment and recovery time.

The following are some possible inquiries to make:

• May I continue to work?

• Can I schedule my chemotherapy for the weekend?

• Should I postpone my vacation?

• Can I travel over the holidays?

• What forms of exercise are secure?

• Should I alter my diet?

You could want assistance with daily tasks while you're receiving treatment and possibly even after you've finished. Invite your close ones to help. Make a list of your unique demands if you think it may help. Hence, family and friends can pick how best to assist.

Below are some areas where you could require assistance:

• Household tasks

• Supermarket shopping

• Consider a Second Opinion

- Walk your dog
- Drive the kids to school
- Prepare meals
- Assist the kids with after-school activities.

• Consider a Second Opinion

You might feel compelled to begin therapy immediately soon. Nonetheless, individuals with early-stage breast cancer typically have some time to process everything. In actuality, you might not be certain of your diagnosis or treatment strategy. Before you make any decisions, it is OK to get a second opinion from a physician.

Get a recommendation for a breast cancer expert. They might concur with your primary physician. Yet, sometimes they might provide you with more options to consider. Be sure the visit is covered by your health insurance by checking with your provider. Request that your doctor email the new doctor all of your medical records.

Life might change after receiving a breast cancer diagnosis. Those close to you will also be impacted. Yet, there are steps you and your loved ones may take to get ready for the future.

Practical Suggestions for Managing Early Breast Cancer

Breast cancer in its early stages is cancer that has not spread to other organs. It is therefore limited to your breasts or the adjacent lymph nodes. Stages I through IIIa and stage 0 ductal carcinoma (milk duct cancer) are included in this.

Early-stage breast cancer can be fought in several effective methods. And you have a good possibility of success. Yet along the road, you'll probably experience some undesirable side effects. The good news is that you can take steps to make treatment and recovery easier. Here are some ideas to get you started.

Consider your future.

Ninety percent of all breast cancer patients will survive five years after receiving treatment. That is the period that is typically utilized to calculate survival rates. If you have stage 1, or breast cancer

that is contained to your breast and has not spread, your 5-year survival rate increases to 99%.
But, it's difficult to predict how cancer will impact you in particular. Your age, general health, the type of cancer you have, as well as other factors, all play a part. Ask your doctor how these factors might affect the outcome of your treatment.

Control hair loss

Chemotherapy and other cancer-fighting medications might harm your hair follicles. Your hair frequently falls out as a result, in part or in full. Certain treatments might just thin out your scalp. But, other medications might have an impact on your pubic hair, arm or leg hair, eyebrows, or eyelashes.

You don't have to be ashamed of your baldness. Many people experience it, and 3 to 5 months following therapy, it typically grows back. But if you're concerned, the following pretreatment advice might be helpful:

• Shorten your hair.

• Inquire with your doctor about using a cooling cap, a device that could slow or stop hair loss.

• Cover your head with a scarf and add a cotton scarf pad for extra bulk.
• Purchase a wig before your therapy begins. The expense of your wig may be covered in whole or in part by your health insurance. So make sure to request a "cranial prosthetic" prescription from your doctor.
If you do start losing hair, take care of your scalp. Extreme sensitivity may result from treatment. To protect your head, you should put on a hat or scarf.
• If you do venture outside in the sun, wear sunscreen with an SPF of 30 or higher.
• Use gentle shampoo and conditioner or baby shampoo.
• Instead of using a brush, use a comb.
• Avoid using flat or curling irons or hair dryers.

Ease Irritation and Vomiting

Cancer treatments frequently leave you feeling ill. Constipation and dehydration are other undesirable side effects that might make you sick.
Ask your doctor whether there are any prescription anti-nausea medications.
• Drink a lot of water unless your doctor directs you otherwise.

• Consider acupressure or acupuncture.
• Consume small meals periodically.
• Choose cold, odorless foods wherever possible.
• When you first get up, have some toast or dry crackers as a snack.
• Have a small snack both before and after chemotherapy.

Furthermore causing nausea is the tension of the procedure. Your sense of calm could increase with relaxation techniques. Deep breathing, yoga, and meditation are examples of common ones. On the back of your neck, you can also place a damp washcloth, either with or without peppermint oil. Wait for 30 minutes before moving it.

Skin and Nail Soothers

Your skin may become red, dry, or irritated from cancer treatment. You may become more sensitive to the sun as a result of radiation therapy. Find out what products to use by asking your cancer care team. They will be aware of which over-the-counter options are soft and mild. They may also recommend the following:
• Use fragrance-free soap and moisturizer.

• Keep underwire bras and tight clothing to a minimum
• Maintain clean skin to avoid infection
• Cover your lips and body with sunscreen with an SPF of 30 or higher.
You might see some changes in your nails. They can split or become discolored. Your cuticles can hurt and bulge. Trim your nails short and moisturize your cuticles and nails with petroleum jelly while the skin is still damp.
Wearing sandals or other looser shoes, not getting manicures or pedicures, and using gloves when doing chores
If DIY solutions don't work, consult your doctor. You could require medical attention for certain skin and nail issues.

Cover up skin blemishes

Your skin's hue can be altered by surgery, chemotherapy, and radiation therapy. You could get spots that are black, red, or appear bruised. After therapy is over, this form of discoloration normally disappears.
You don't need to conceal skin changes because they are common. Yet if you conceal the uneven areas,

you might feel more like yourself. Before using cosmetics like concealer or foundation, especially if you have a rash, see your cancer care team. You can get advice from your doctor on the best things to use while undergoing treatment.

Update Your Clothes

You could not be thinking about fashion at all. However, there are many ways that cancer treatment might impact your health. Physically and emotionally painful, these adjustments can be. The following items can potentially lessen adverse effects and improve your self-esteem.

Put comfort first. Throughout treatment, you might gain or lose weight. And you can get extremely sensitive skin. Choose clothing that will enable you to adapt to the situation, such as loose-fitting tops or dresses, cotton clothing, or pants or skirts with an elastic waist.

Camisoles in exchange for an underwire. You can get support from these gentle clothes without your skin being overly stressed.

Buy breast cancer apparel. Many fashion companies design their products with healing and therapy in

mind. Make a quick web search to discover what is available. Examples of what you might discover are as follows:
• Robes, tanks, camisoles, or hoodies with easy access to a port-a-cath, as well as soft loungewear without seams
• Shirts or hoodies with surgical drain storage
• Undies for breast reconstruction or post-surgery

Intimacy and Sex

Your sex life might change as a result of breast cancer treatment. Since you're exhausted or don't like the way your body appears, you might not be as in the mood. It's crucial to express your feelings to your mate. You may decide how they can help you the most effectively by working together. Speak with your doctor as well. For example, they can assist in treating vaginal dryness. Also, a therapist or support group can assist you in resolving additional issues with intimacy and sex.

Conclusion

Breast cancer is caused by multiple causes, many of which may act alone or in combination, especially in high-risk individuals. Knowing the pathophysiology of this widespread illness, which is linked to high mortality and morbidity rates, is crucial, especially if it is not caught early. To detect recurrence at an early stage, it has been suggested that early screening in high-risk persons as well as adequate surveillance of treated cases be used.

Finding out you have breast cancer can be frightening, annoying, and even hopeless. Perhaps you or your loved one is suffering with this illness, it's critical that you take advantage of the many resources that are offered to you. With your healthcare provider, go over your treatment options. Before making a choice, you might even want to seek out a second opinion. Your treatment strategy should make you happy and upbeat. Also, talking with others who are experiencing the same thing might help with feelings of loneliness, so consider attending a local support group.